A Simple Bone Broth Recipe To Heal Leaky Gut Syndrome

OLOXIR

ISBN: 1544774761
ISBN-13: 978-1544774763

CONTENTS MAIN

Introduction

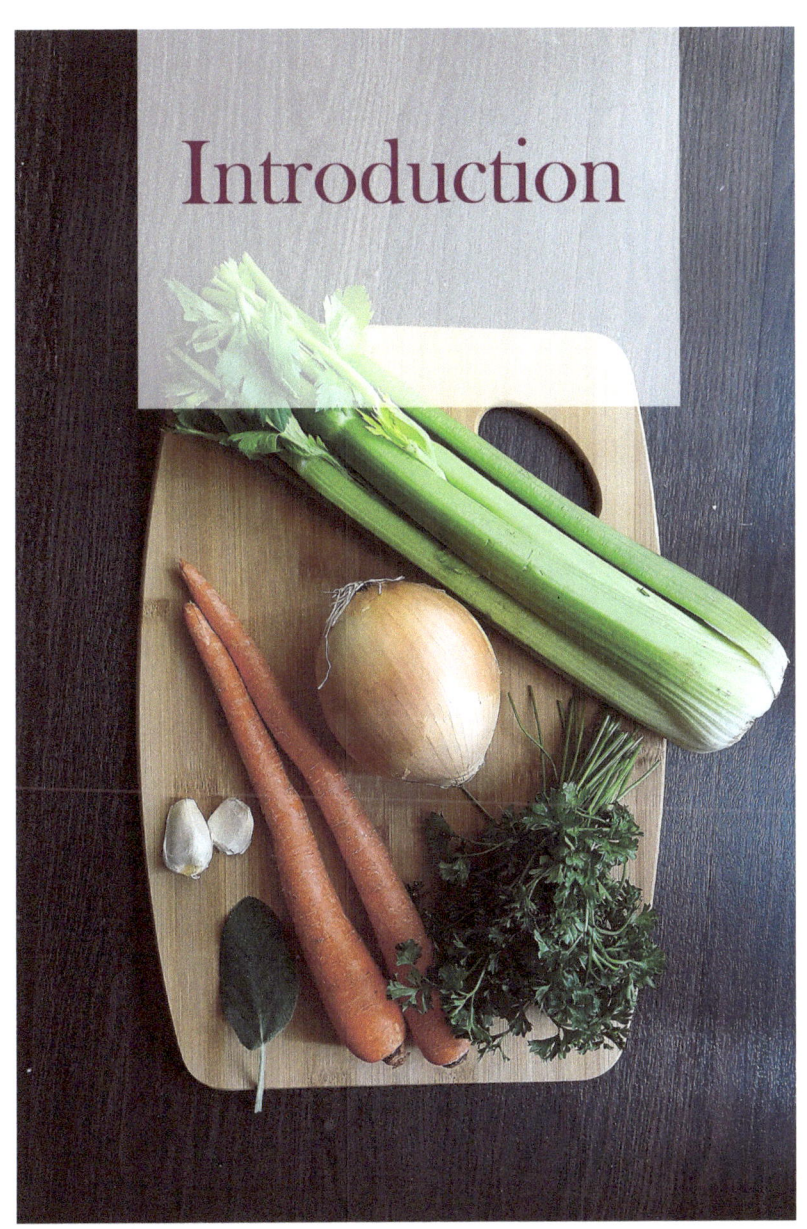

INTRODUCTION

I remember the first day I began making bone broth. Impressed by its gut health benefits, I rushed to the store and picked out a meaty beef soup bone, onion, celery, carrots and garlic cloves to throw in for flavor.

After sprinkling the bones with vinegar, I added the water and let the broth simmer happily away. But what happened next is probably predictable. It was about three hours in and while sitting on the sofa I began to smell the most delicious aroma of meat and onions.

Wait. *Why am I smelling onions?*

I jumped from the sofa and bolted into the kitchen. Sure enough, my bone broth had cooked down to nothingness *minus* what the now browning onions had absorbed. I don't need to elaborate on the disappointment that ensued.

But I'm not one to give up. Since then, I've graduated to making tasty bone broth on a weekly basis and so can you. In addition to going over the gut healing benefits that bone broth provides, I am going to show you what I wish I knew as a beginner so that you get it right *without* burning the onions. We will cover everything from prep and techniques to cooking, storing and adding flavor. Let's begin by addressing how bone broth can help heal a leaky gut.

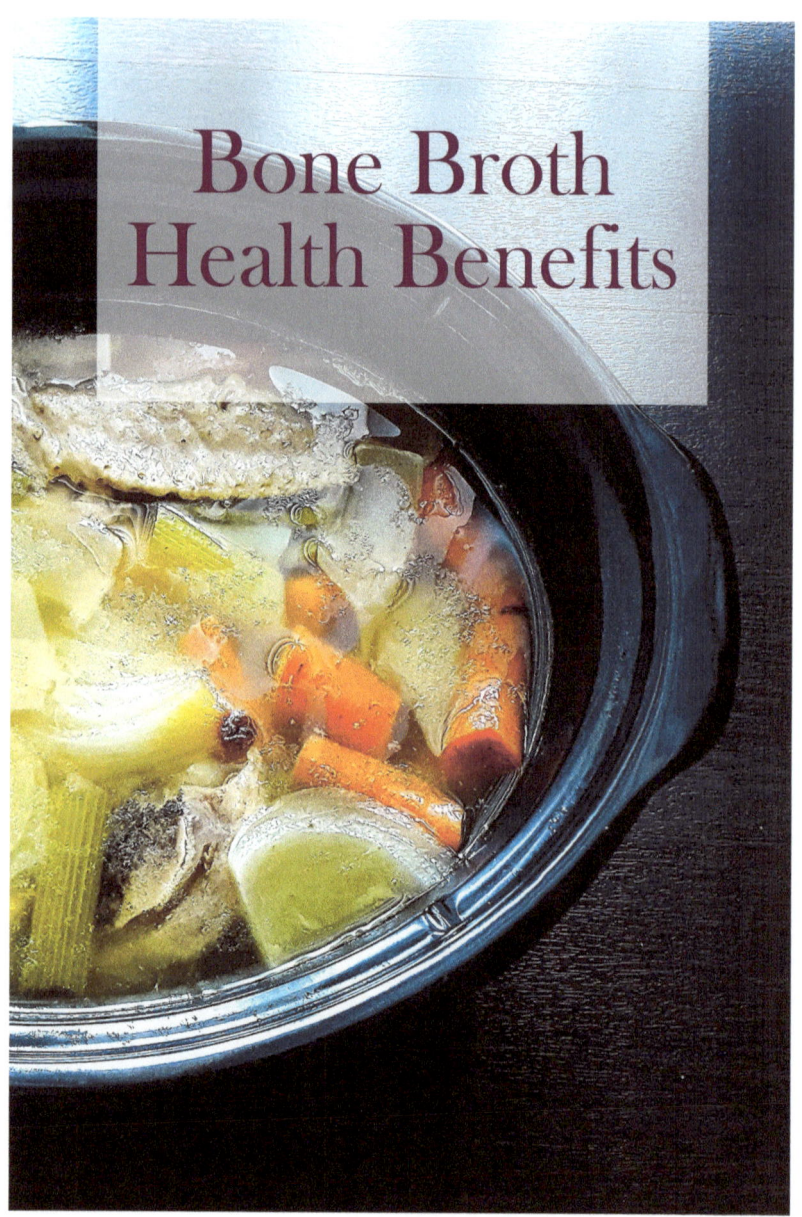

Bone Broth
Health Benefits

1 BONE BROTH HEALTH BENEFITS

Bone broth is packed amino acids like Glutamine, Glycine, Proline, Arginine, and Cysteine. Sound good? Homemade bone broth is also an excellent source of collagen and nourishing minerals. Let's take a quick look at the benefits each of these can provide. This will help you better understand the role bone broth plays in healing a Leaky Gut.

Glutamine
Glutamine is a key amino acid required by cells in the intestines to function efficiently and absorb the nutrients from your food. Stress reduces glutamine levels and when the intestinal cells don't get enough of this amino acid, their ability to prevent pathogens from leaking into the body is also reduced. This is why getting enough glutamine is pivotal for healing a Leaky Gut and bone broth is an excellent source.

Glycine

Glycine is another amino acid found in bone broth that greatly benefits the gut. How? When it comes to digestion, glycine aids in the healthy production of bile and stomach acid required to properly digest food. Glycine also nourishes the liver and helps our body to create glutathione. Furthermore, glutathione works as an antioxidant[1] to prevent damage to our cells and neutralize free radicals -both important for good health.

Proline

Proline is an imino acid (yes, imino[2]) that is essential for producing cartilage and collagen. Joints and muscles also benefit from the flexibility that proline provides. Found in bone broth, proline is a fundamental component that aids in repairing the intestinal lining and healing a leaky gut.

Arginine

Arginine is an amino acid with anti-inflammatory properties. It's essential for a healthy immune system and plays an important role in the healing of wounds. Arginine also works alongside proline to heal the intestinal lining.

---

[1] http://www.medicinenet.com/script/main/art.asp?articlekey=50746

[2] http://www.biology.arizona.edu/biochemistry/problem_sets/aa/proline.html

Cysteine

Remember the glutathione we mentioned earlier? Cysteine is essential for its production. This amino acid is also necessary for the healthy appearance of nails, skin and hair.

Health Benefits of the Collagen Found in Bone Broth

Speaking of beautiful hair, skin and nails -next up is collagen. Collagen improves the absorption of nutrients, reduces the appearance of wrinkles and combats cellulite. The best part? Bone broth is cheaper than your anti-aging cream.

In the Journal of Clinical Gastroenterology, a report showed that **gelatin**, a water-soluble protein derived from collagen, helps to maintain the health and structure of your intestines. A bone broth that jiggles once cooled is the trademark of gelatin and this exactly what you are aiming for when making your own bone broth at home. Utilizing neck and joint bones in your broth will help you to achieve this result, but more on that later.

Collagen also contains two amino acids from above – **proline** and **glycine**, which helps to prevent inflammatory conditions such as heartburn or gastroesophageal reflux disease (GERD).

Health Benefits of the Minerals Found in

Bone Broth

Magnesium, potassium, phosphorus, silica, calcium and even iodine can be found in bones. These same nutrients can be extracted and consumed as bone broth. Working together, they help keep the body hydrated and contribute to healthy cell function and bones. Adding an acidic element like vinegar will help maximize the extraction of these nutrients from the broth. We'll cover how to do this in detail.

The Bottom Line...

Bone broth is low in calories, packed with essential and non-essential vitamins, contains collagen and gelatin which is good for the gut. It also provides nutrients essential for easy digestion, bolsters the immune system and a whole lot more – easy to see why this natural food is beneficial to the body.

Choosing The Best Bones

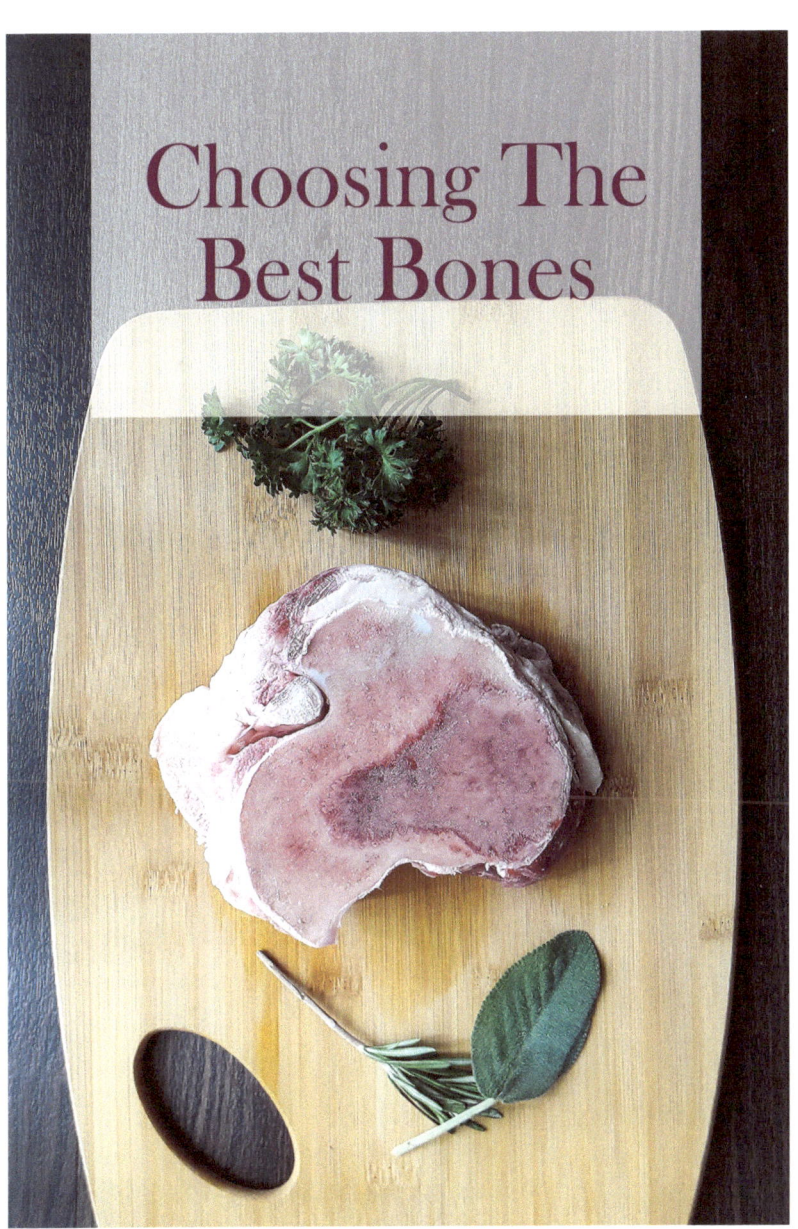

2 CHOOSING THE BEST BONES

It goes without saying that you can't make bone broth without the bones. But as a beginner, you may be wondering which bones are best and how to get a hold of them. Thankfully, bone broth can be made from practically any type of bone. However, for best results and to get that nourishing collagen, you will want to add in either marrow, neck or knuckle bones. I find that by tossing in a few neck bones (chicken, pork and even lamb) I consistently get a bone broth that gels. Another plus? Neck bones are also more affordable than marrow bones in most grocery stores.

Good Bones

A healthy, nourishing broth begins with a healthy animal. This is non-negotiable. If you cannot obtain bones from grass fed animals, you still have options. Look for bones from animals that are raised on a healthy diet *without* antibiotics, additives etc. Information such as this is typically stated on the packaging.

Chicken Bones

Chicken bones are a great place to start if you are beginner to bone broth. Organic chicken is readily accessible and your eyes will recognize the bones as familiar territory. Save the meat for a meal and toss the rest into the pot to simmer for at least 12 hours.

If you have access to friends or a farmer that raises chicken for meat in your area, ask them what they do with the bones. This can be a cheaper way of getting organic bones for next to nothing, or at the very least cheaper than most grocers.

Turkey Bones

Turkey bones work equally as well. If you are using a whole turkey carcass, then you will want to use a larger pot to accommodate the bones. This will yield a bigger batch of broth, but again you can strain and store the broth in the freezer until you are ready to consume it. Buying a whole turkey is usually reserved to once a year on Thanksgiving for most of us. So if you want to make a smaller batch, you can find turkey breasts, backs, legs, wings and necks at the grocer. I often add in a turkey back, wings or turkey neck to help the bone

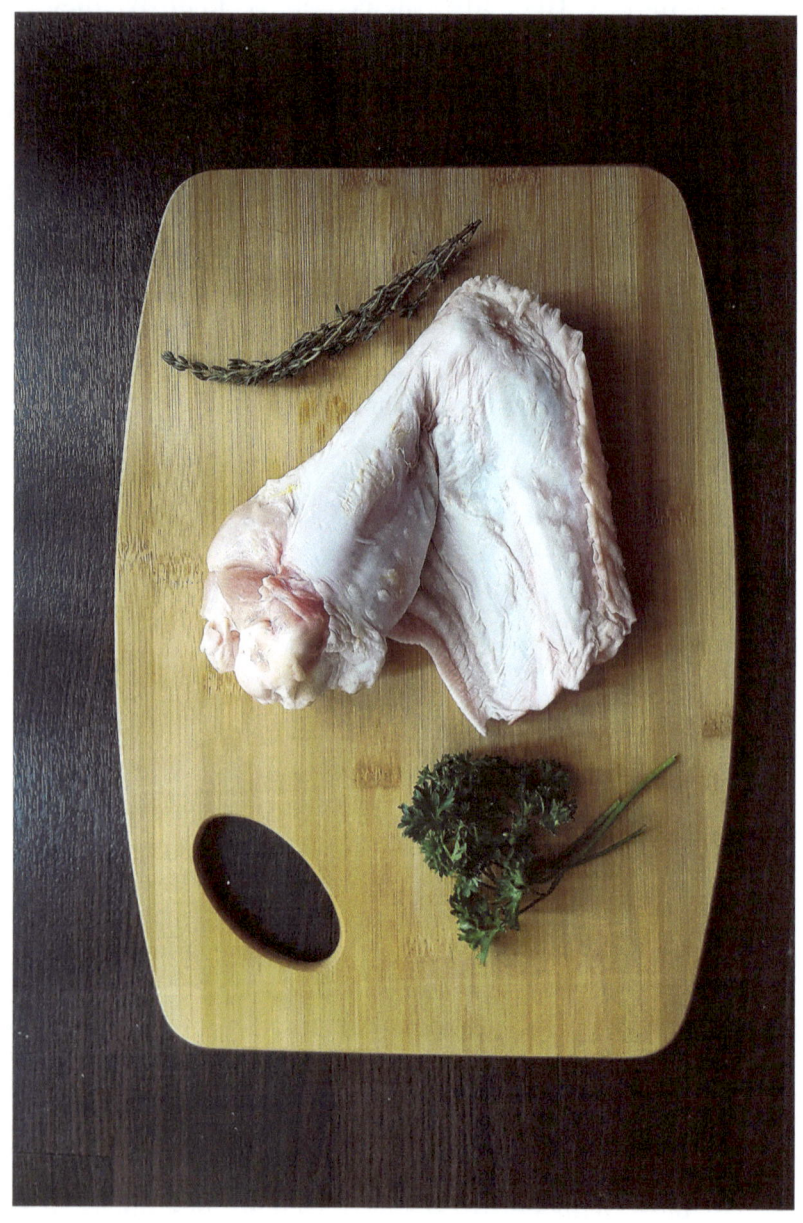

broth gel, and the cost is next to nothing.

Beef, Pork and Lamb Bones

Beef bones are my favorite base for creating a good, tasty broth. But due to their popularity, I have to get to the store early to grab some before they sell out. Here is where having a relationship with your local butcher will come in handy.

Roasting beef, lamb or pork bones before you make the broth will give you a rich flavor and beautiful color. To do this, preheat your oven to 450 F.

Arrange the bones in a single layer on a baking sheet and roast for 20 to 25 minutes. Allow the bones to cool so that you can safely handle them. Then proceed to add to the pot with apple cider vinegar and water. Broth using these bones should simmer for a minimum of 18 hours. I love to use beef soup bones a base and then add in a few marrow, poultry, lamb or pork bones.

Lamb adds a wonderful depth to the flavor of your bone broth and funny enough, when I add pork bones the broth has a hint of breakfast sausage flavor -seriously. This is your bone broth, so blend the bones as you choose.

Vegetables & Herbs

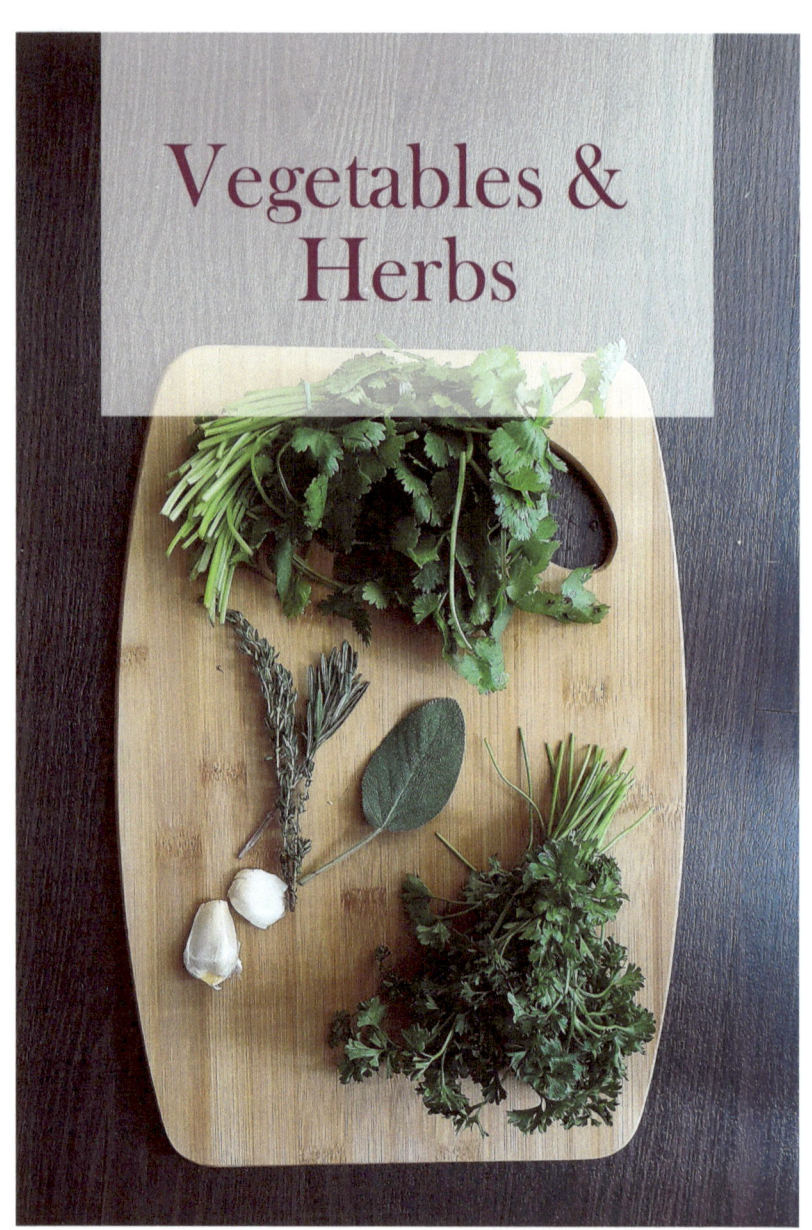

3 VEGETABLES & HERBS

Once you have the bone broth basics down, you'll want to shake things up a bit by introducing new flavors. The best part about making your own homemade bone broth is that you can mix in anything that suits your palate. In the land of black and white, you, my friend, are a vibrant red. Spice up your bone broth accordingly.

There are a few ways that you can go about accomplishing this. You can add your favorite aromatics, seasonings and vegetables during the cooking process or simply add a handful of herbs at the end of the cooking process. In fact, by adding your herbs and seasoning at the end of the cooking process you can tweak the flavor of the broth depending on who's eating it. Something as simple as a pinch of salt, pepper, chives or fresh rosemary can be added up serving for an extra punch of flavor to individual servings.

Making a basic bone broth will also give you added flexibility when it comes to using your broth in other recipes. A neutral flavor is easier to blend into soups, rice and even smoothies (yes, people do this). Keeping things basic adds a depth of flavor that doesn't over power the dish, so always season your broth with the end goal in mind. Let's go over popular vegetables, herbs and spices that make delicious additions for elevating the flavor profile of your bone broth.

The Usual Suspects
Salt
Pepper
Green Onion

Vegetables
Carrots
Celery
Onion
Leeks
Tomato

Fresh or Dried Herbs
Garlic
Parsley
Basil
Oregano
Rosemary
Sage

Chive
Thyme

Spices
Cayenne
Turmeric
Curry
Cumin
Soy Sauce

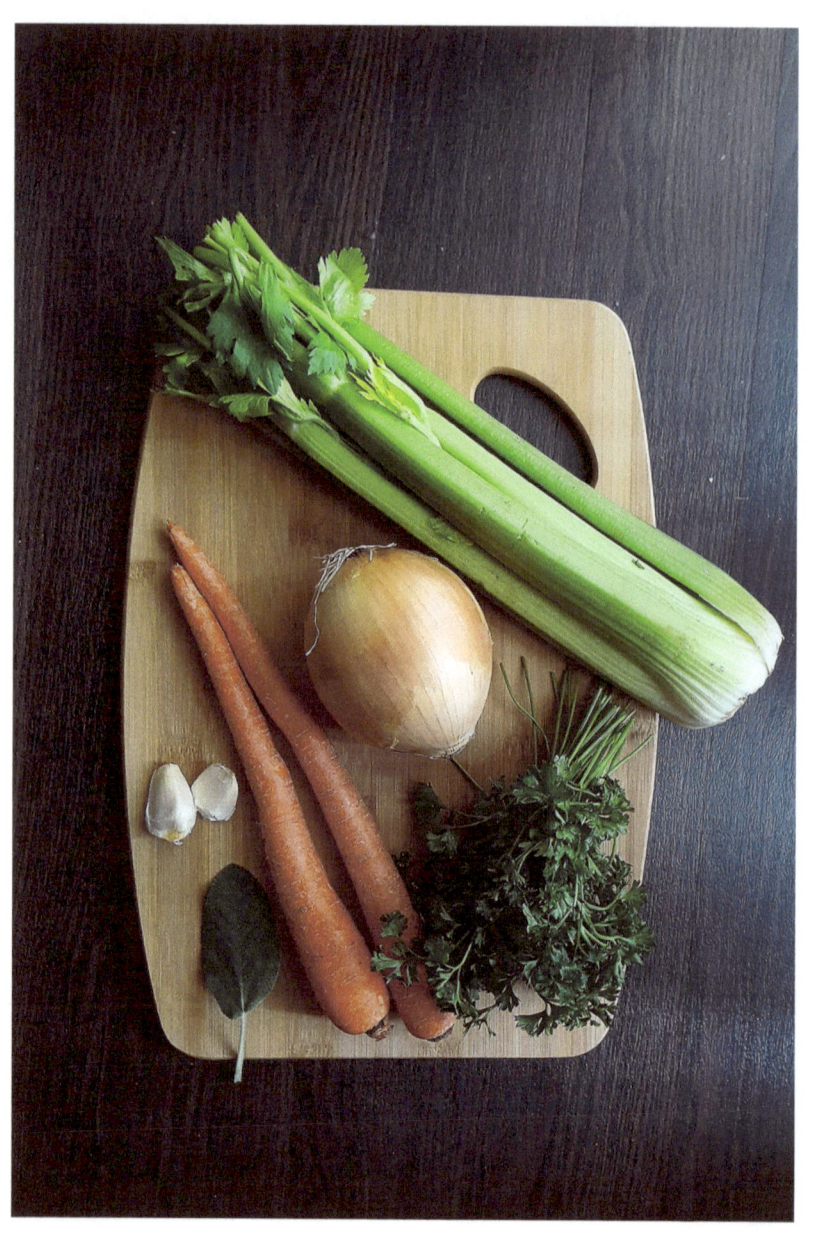

This is not an all-inclusive list. If there is a spice or vegetable that you enjoy, try adding it into your bone broth for additional flavor.

When it comes to adding these flavor additions, timing is important. For example, if you add vegetables at the beginning by the time your bone broth completes the flavor, along with everything else, will have cooked out. A rule of thumb is to add your vegetables around 6 hours before the bone broth is complete. So, if you are making a 12-hour bone broth, add the vegetables 6 hours into cook time. The 6-hour window gives enough time for the nutrients to be extracted into the broth without compromising flavor.

It's okay to add dried spices and herbs at the beginning; however, when it comes to using fresh herbs you will want to wait until the end of the cooking process to add them. Again, if you add them at the beginning, you will lose the benefits and flavor. If you want the flavor to cook in a bit, then add the fresh herbs one hour before cook time ends. So, if you are making a 12-hour broth, add the fresh herbs 11 hours into cook time. Alternatively, simply add them at the end for a fresh burst of flavor.

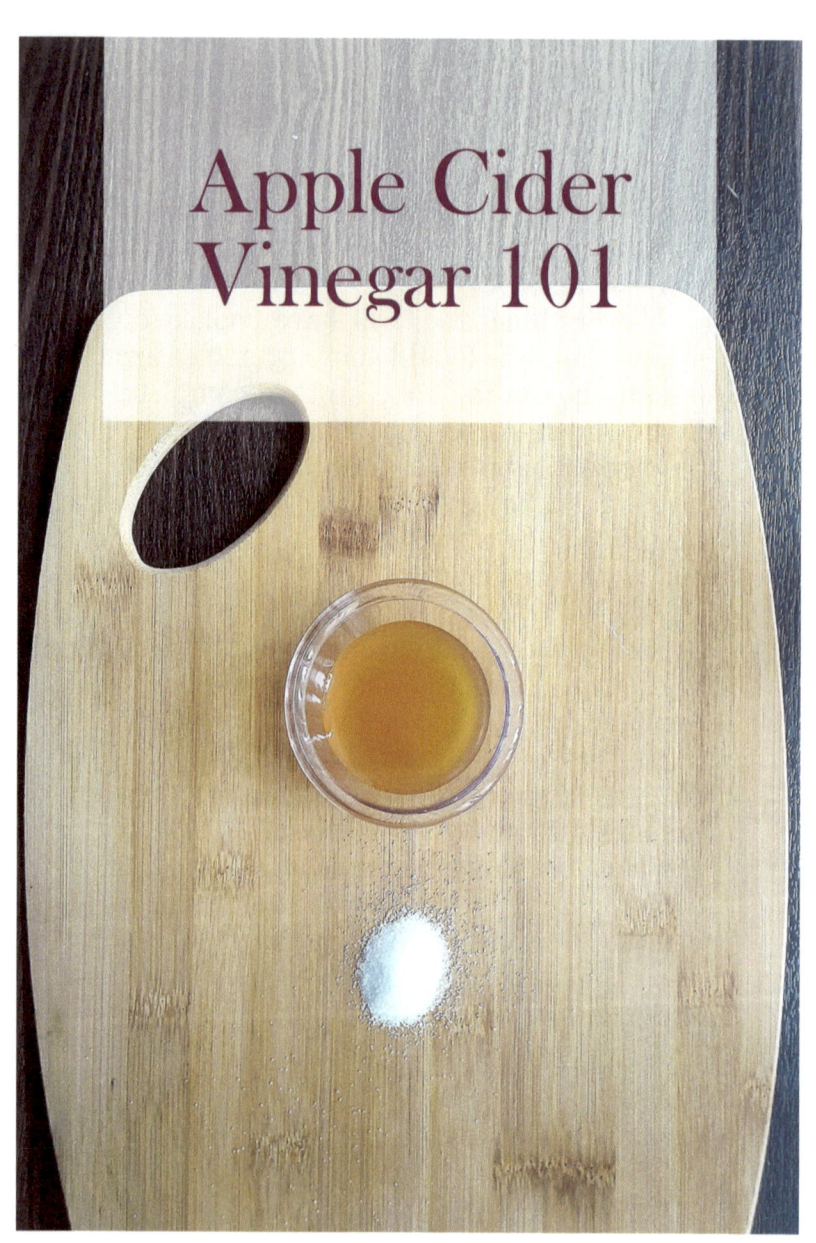

Apple Cider Vinegar 101

4 APPLE CIDER VINEGAR 101

Look at any bone broth recipe and you will see apple cider vinegar as part of the ingredient list. There is an excellent reason for this. Including apple cider vinegar to your bone broth adds to the nutritional and health benefits you gain from sipping this savory broth. Let's go into a little more detail on why you should be adding apple cider vinegar to your crock pot.

Get More Minerals from Your Broth

The number one reason to add apple cider vinegar to your bone broth to extract more of the minerals and nutrients from the bones. The acidity of apple cider vinegar helps to pull minerals such as potassium, calcium and magnesium from the bones and into your broth.

One of the greatest health benefits of bone broth is its density of nutrients and minerals that we just don't get enough of in the modern day diet. Maximize the health benefits of your bone broth by adding apple cider vinegar to the pot when preparing your broth. If you don't have apple cider vinegar handy, plain white vinegar will also get the job done.

It's A Preservative

The next reason why you will want to add apple cider vinegar is that it functions as a preservative. The acidic nature of the apple cider vinegar will eliminate bacteria and keep your cooked bone broth safe to consume. It's very similar to how pickling helps to preserve produce.

With that said, apple cider vinegar is not the end of all solution to safety. There isn't enough power in the apple cider vinegar to kill everything. This is why you should immediately store your bone broth in the refrigerator or in the freezer once it has cooled.

Why Apple Cider Vinegar

So, why apple cider vinegar? Well, any type of vinegar will help to pull out the nutrients from the bones and act as a preservative. However, apple cider vinegar provides added benefits when it comes to digestion. Organic, unpasteurized apple cider vinegar is packed with gut healthy bacteria. It also contains essential amino acids and active yeast. As you can see, apple cider vinegar gives your bone broth an added health boost that plain white vinegar simply cannot deliver.

Where to Get Apple Cider Vinegar

Quality apple cider vinegar can be found at local health foods stores and even in most major supermarkets. When it comes to organic, unpasteurized apple cider vinegar Bragg's is a popular and affordable brand.

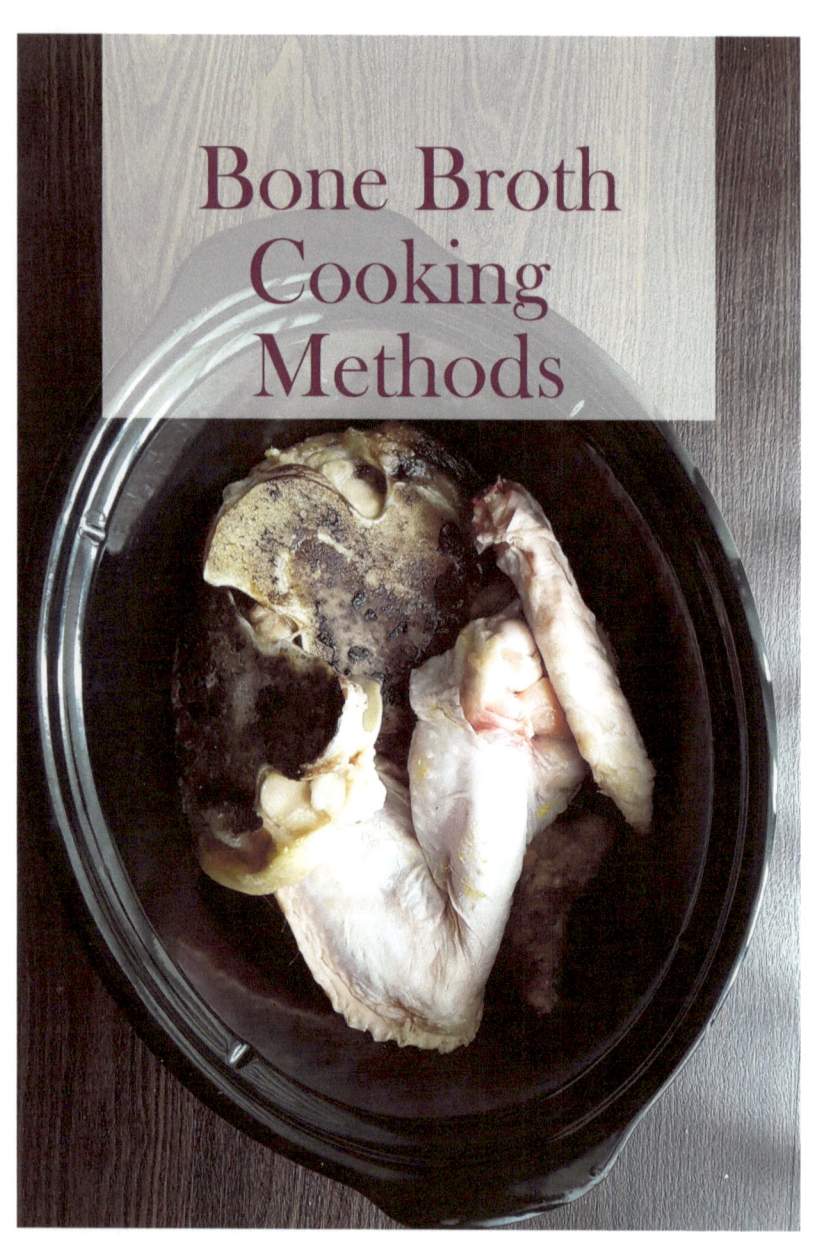

Bone Broth Cooking Methods

5 BONE BROTH COOKING METHODS

Like many things, bone broth gets better with time. The longer you simmer the bones, the greater the flavor and nutritional benefits. Again, the minimum you want to cook your broth for is 12 hours for chicken and at least 18 hours for other meats. If you're of the "go big or go home" mentality, you're looking at a 48 to 72 hours simmer.

This can be challenging for those with a busy lifestyle but I've found 24 hours using a crockpot to be a very happy medium. There are three main techniques for cooking bone broth. All of which we will go over in detail shortly, but in short you'll use a stock pot on the burner, utilize a crockpot, or make a perpetual broth that continually cooks and you dip into it as needed.

All three methods will yield the same result

so it really comes down to your personal preference. If you are going to be at home throughout the day, stove top cooking will work just fine. If you've got to work or prefer to simmer overnight, then a crockpot will be a better option for you.

Begin with the easiest option as this will ensure your long term success. For example, I make a crockpot batch once a week and then store the bone broth (I will show you how to do this) for daily use during the week. If I had to use the stock pot method, this would not be possible due to my schedule. So, again -choose the method that works best for you.

Stock Pot Method

Stock pot bone broth is the most traditional way of cooking the broth. Think medieval fires in the long hall with blackened pots bubbling away. Due to the large size of a stock pot, you will be able to make a larger batch without cramming too many bones into the pot. Here's how.

Grab your stock pot and place the bones for your broth inside. If they still have a bit of meat or cartilage left on them, don't worry. It's fine. You actually want some cartilage as it will break down and add create a gelatin that's soothing for your joints and gut. Next up, add the apple cider vinegar and water.

Place the lid on the stock pot and bring the water to a boil. Then, reduce the heat to a simmer and let the bone broth cook for 12 to 72 hours. Begin your broth early in the morning on a day that you know you will be home. Simmer the broth throughout the day until it's time for you to go to bed. Turn the heat off and sleep with peace of mind that you're not burning the house down.

When you wake up in the morning, return the broth to a boil and then continue to simmer during the day. Repeat until you reach your desired cook time. Again, the longer you simmer the bone broth, the better the end result.

When the bone broth is cooked for the desired duration, strain the liquid and store in the refrigerator for three to four days. If you've made too much to be consumed in four days, don't worry. The rest can be frozen and kept for up to a year.

Crock Pot Method

If the above sounds like too much of a hassle, another excellent alternative is to use a crockpot. Especially for smaller batches. I find that a 6-quart crock pot yields around 7-8 one cup servings of bone broth.

Start by placing your bones in the crockpot. Then, sprinkle them with apple cider vinegar as this will help to draw the minerals and other nutrients from the bones. Then turn your crockpot on low and let the bone broth simmer away as long as desired. When using a crockpot, I have simmered for both 18 hours and 24 hours. Both time frames yielded a delicious broth.

Perpetual Method

The third technique for making bone broth is called a perpetual bone broth. In short, you have pot of broth that is continually simmering. You take out what you want to sip or cook with, then add more water and bones as needed to keep the broth going.

This is often done by placing the pot out of the way on the back burner and then turning it off at night. Again, this would work if you are home all the time, but if not, opt for the safety and peace of mind of a crockpot.

A perpetual broth is most handy when you or others in your household are sick. It's a good way to get a continual supply of hot broth without too much effort. To begin a perpetual broth, add the bones to the pot or crockpot along with desired flavorings. Next, cover with water and cook for at least 12 hours.

After you hit the 12-hour mark, you can start dipping into the bone broth as needed. Just be sure to replace the liquid that you take out with water. After 3 days, you will want to either freeze or discard remaining broth and begin again.

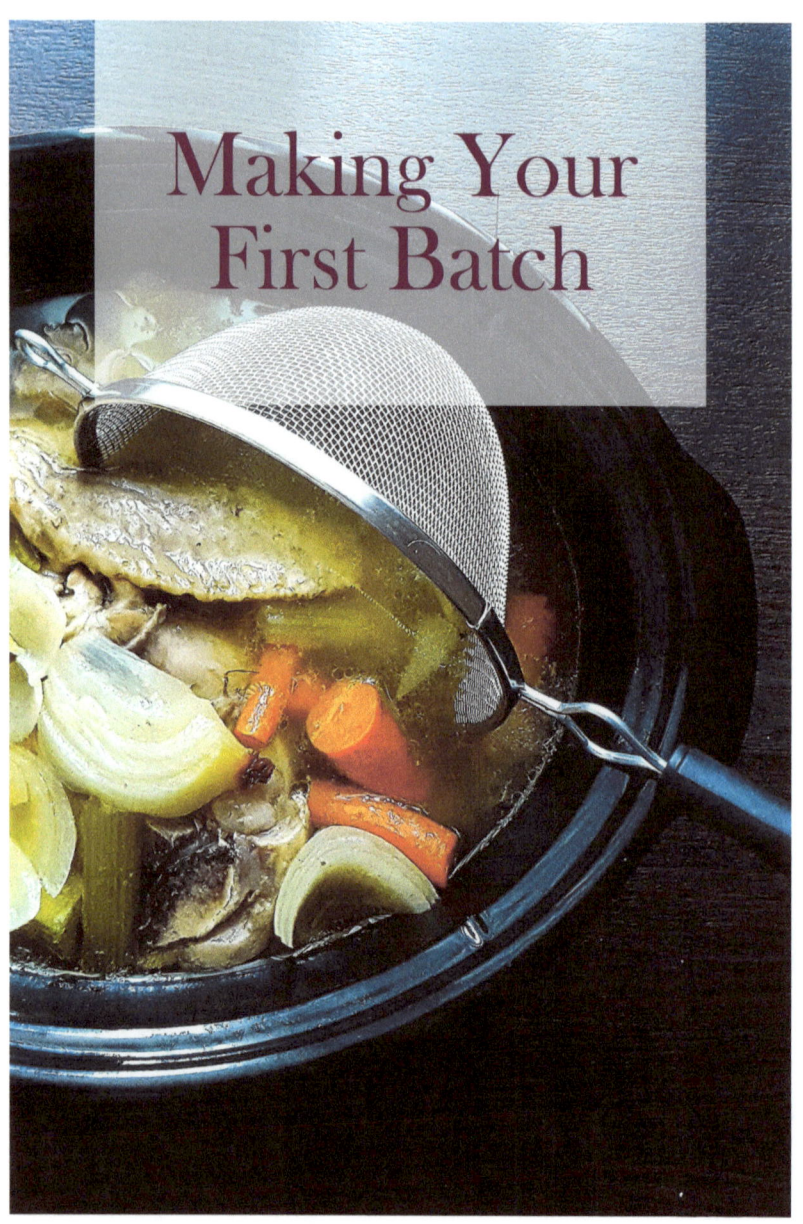

Making Your First Batch

6 MAKING YOUR FIRST BATCH

Bone broth is the nourishing end result of boiling bones from poultry, beef or pork in water for an extended amount of time. While delicious sipped from a mug on its own, bone broth can also add a nutritional punch to stews, soups and other foods. Unlike the broth that most of us are familiar with, bone broth requires a longer cook time to release the health benefits it's known for.

Simmering the bones for a long period of time allows them to break down and release multiple nutrients, minerals, collagen and glucosamine. In fact, this nutritional value is exactly why people cook and consume bone broth on a regular basis.

When it comes to making bone broth for the first time, there are two ways to go about it. Either start with cooked meat or pick up bones from your local butcher or store. If you are starting with cooked meat, say a chicken that you have roasted or purchased from the grocery store, here's what you will want to do. Remove all the cooked meat of the chicken and set aside. This is your dinner. Leftovers? Add the chicken meat to the bone broth you are about to create for a delicious soup.

After all the edible meat has been removed, place the bones and any extra bits of meat you didn't sneak to the dog into the pot. If you decided to start with store bought bones, soak them in cool water for about 20min. This mini bath helps to remove the blood from the bones that's usually present when you take them out of the packaging. Then place the bones in the pot.

Next, you will want to drizzle a few tablespoons of apple cider vinegar over the bones. Again, the apple cider vinegar helps to pull the minerals out of the bones and into your bone broth. If you don't have apple cider vinegar handy, it's okay to substitute with white vinegar.

Finally, add your water as per the recipe. While adding more water will yield more broth, too much water will minimize our chances of getting a good gel when the broth cools. Cover your pot with a lid and bring to a boil. Then you will want to reduce the heat to a simmer.

Chicken bone broth should be cooked for a minimum of 12 hours and beef or pork bone broth for a minimum of 18 hours. For maximum benefits, bone broth can be cooked for up to 48 hours. For obvious reasons, be sure to only simmer the broth on the stove when you are fully awake and inside of the house.

Six hours before cook time ends, add your vegetables to the broth. Cover and continue simmering until desired cook time is reached. Again, fresh herbs can be added up to an hour before cook time is complete or afterwards.

If you've made a large batch of bone broth, more likely than not you will have more broth than you can possibly consume before it goes bad. You will want to freeze what you won't be using within the next 3 to 4 days for later use. Bone broth can be stored in glass jars or plastic container and then placed into the freezer for storage. To use, simply take down and thaw bone broth portions as you need them. After making a batch of bone broth, I usually place 3 one cup servings in the fridge and then

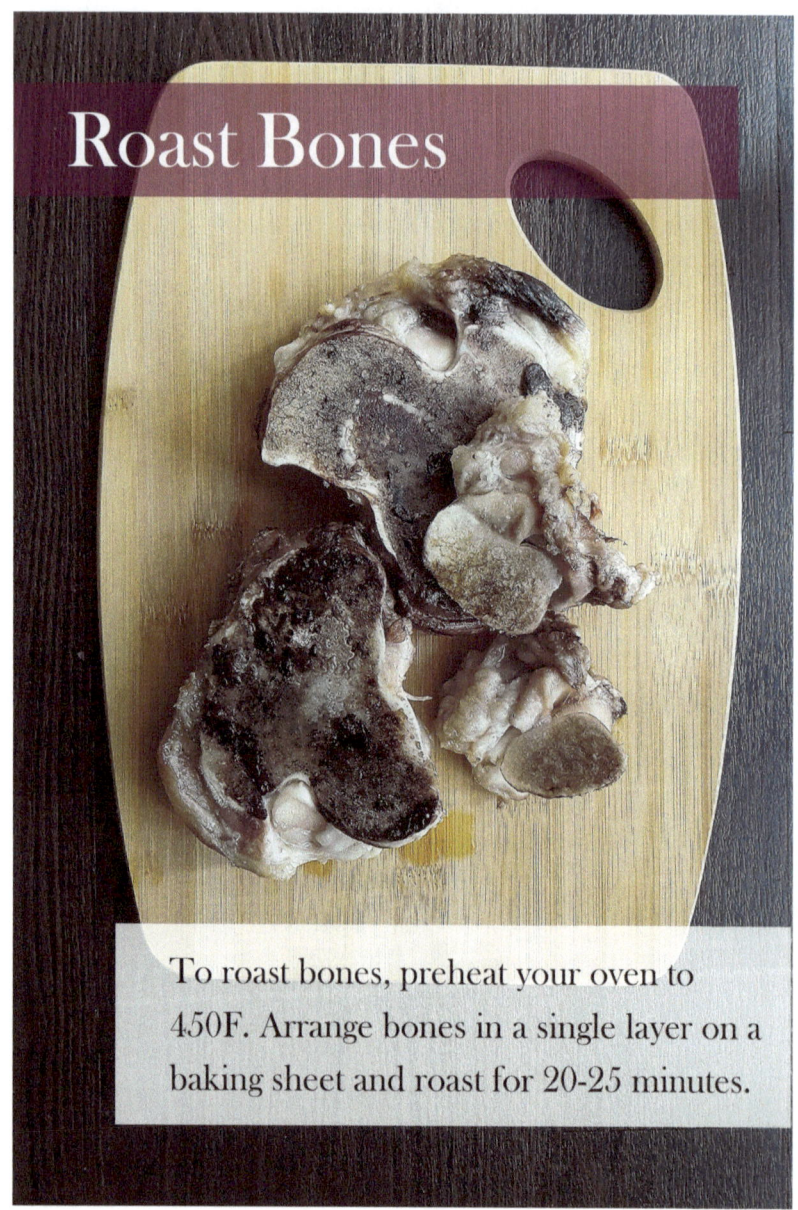

Roast Bones

To roast bones, preheat your oven to 450F. Arrange bones in a single layer on a baking sheet and roast for 20-25 minutes.

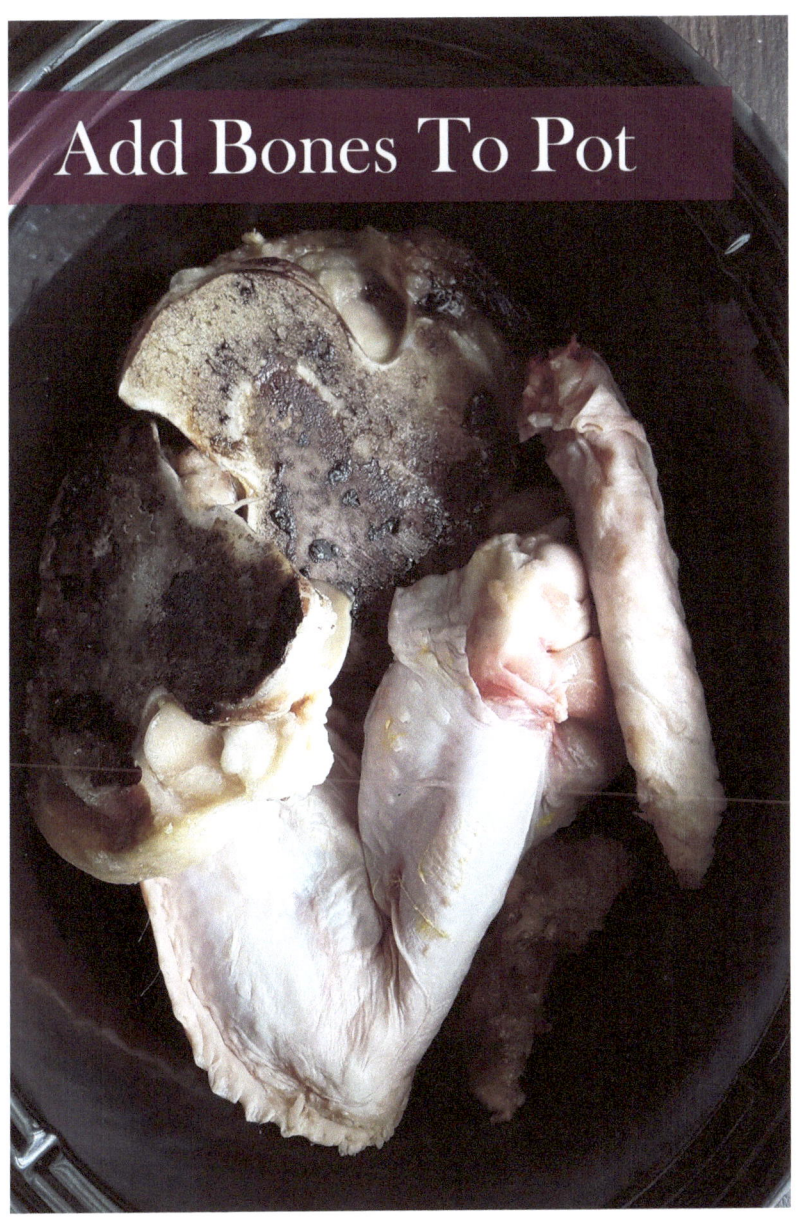

Add Bones To Pot

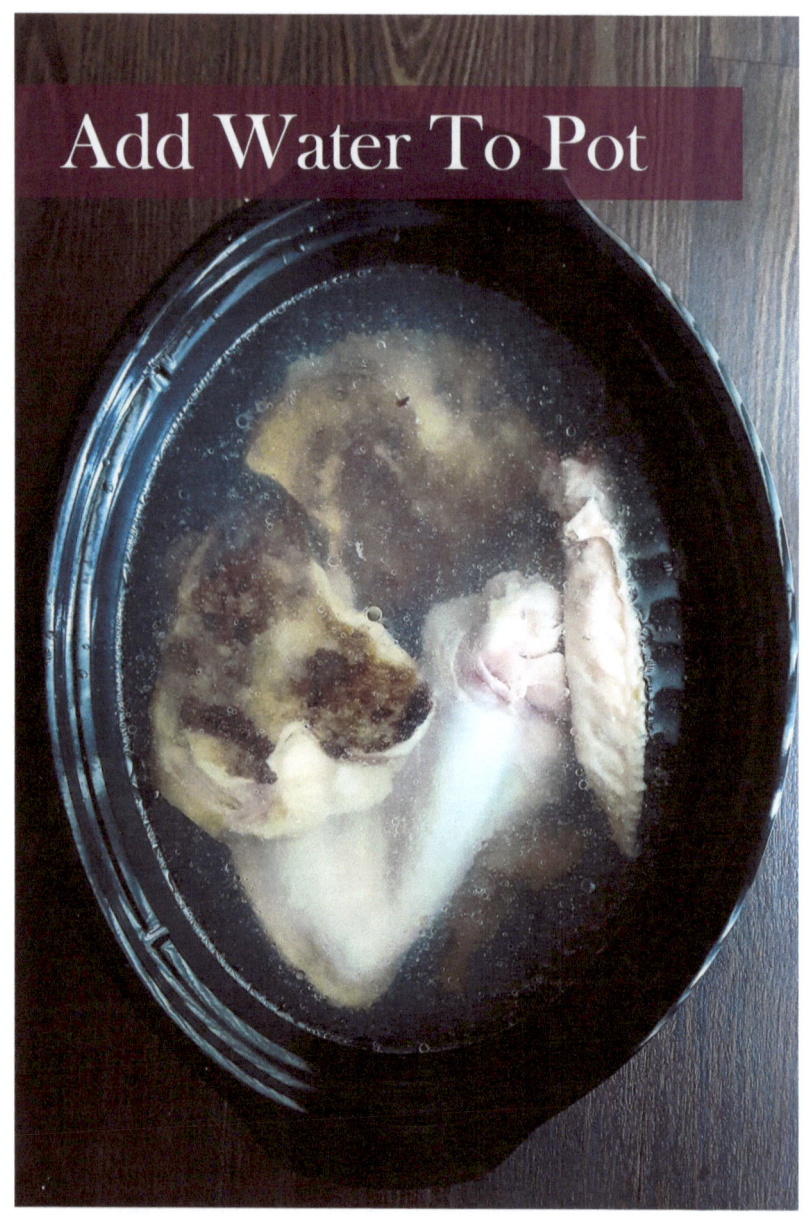

Add Water To Pot

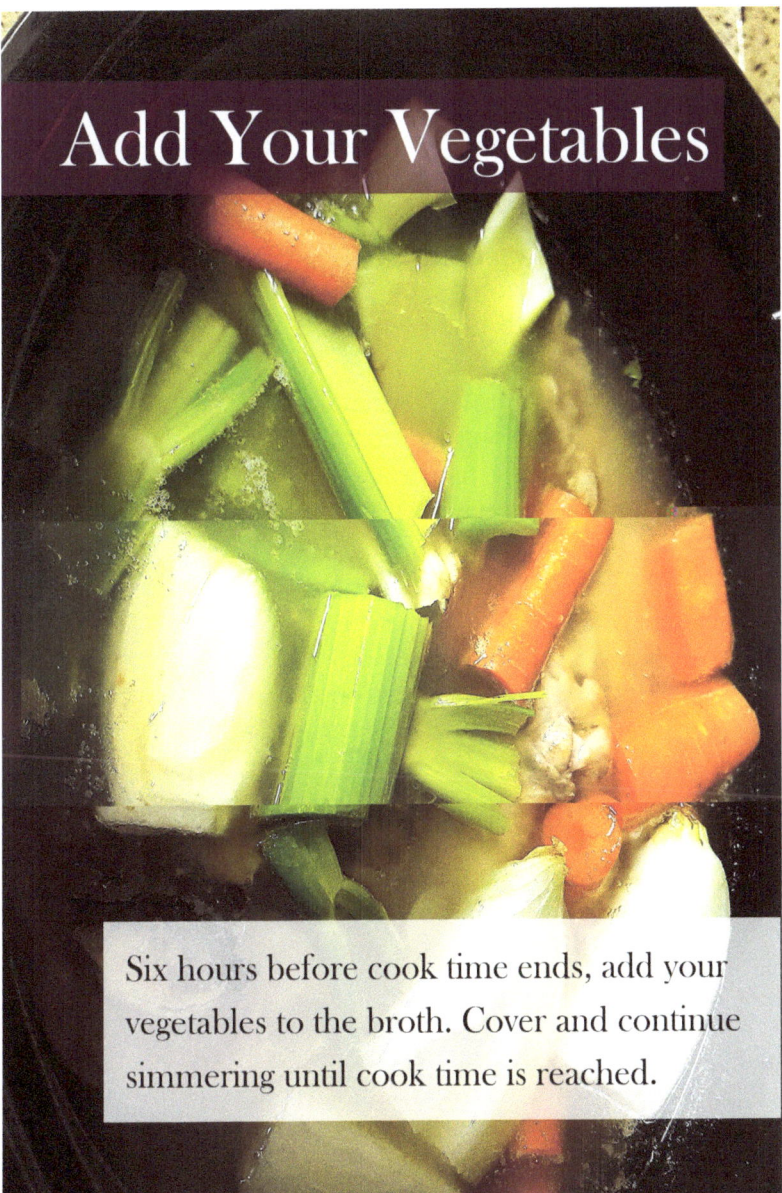

Add Your Vegetables

Six hours before cook time ends, add your vegetables to the broth. Cover and continue simmering until cook time is reached.

If you've made a large batch of bone broth, more likely than not you will have more broth than you can possibly consume before it goes bad. You will want to freeze what you won't be using within the next 3 to 4 days for later use. Bone broth can be stored in glass jars or plastic container and then placed into the freezer for storage. To use, simply take down and thaw bone broth portions as you need them. After making a batch of bone broth, I usually place 3 one cup servings in the fridge and then freeze individual one cup servings in small freezer bags. This makes it easy for me and those in my household to only use what we need, without spoiling the rest.

Another thing you can do is freeze your bone broth in an ice cube tray. Once the bone broth cubes are frozen, pop them out and put them in a freezer bag. When cooking, you can add a couple of cubes to your dish for added nutrition and flavor. This works particularly well with vegetables.

In addition to sipping on warm bone broth, you can also use it as a substitute for store bought broth or stock cubes. As previously mentioned, bone broth makes a delicious base for stews and soups. Instead of using water or stock cubes, use your homemade bone broth instead. It's also a good cheat to add a home-cooked flavor to prepared meals.

Another favorite is to use bone broth to cook

your rice instead of plain water. It tastes really good and the nutritional benefit is always a plus. Same goes for pasta. After cooking your pasta in the broth, serve the broth as a starter at the beginning of the meal.

Beans are a household favorite and replacing even just a cup of the water with broth results in a great pot of beans without the extra ham or bacon. I've tried using broth with and without bacon and the both options are flavorful. And if dairy is something that you are avoiding, whip your mashed potatoes with bone broth instead of milk for a savory side dish. While you're at it, use some bone broth for your gravy to top it off.

While this is not related to cooking, bone broth also makes a great post-work out drink. I found that after consuming bone broth daily for a few weeks, I no longer experienced the pain in my knees after a workout that I did previously. It's great for helping your body to rehydrate and provides a boost thanks to the vitamins, minerals and amino acids.

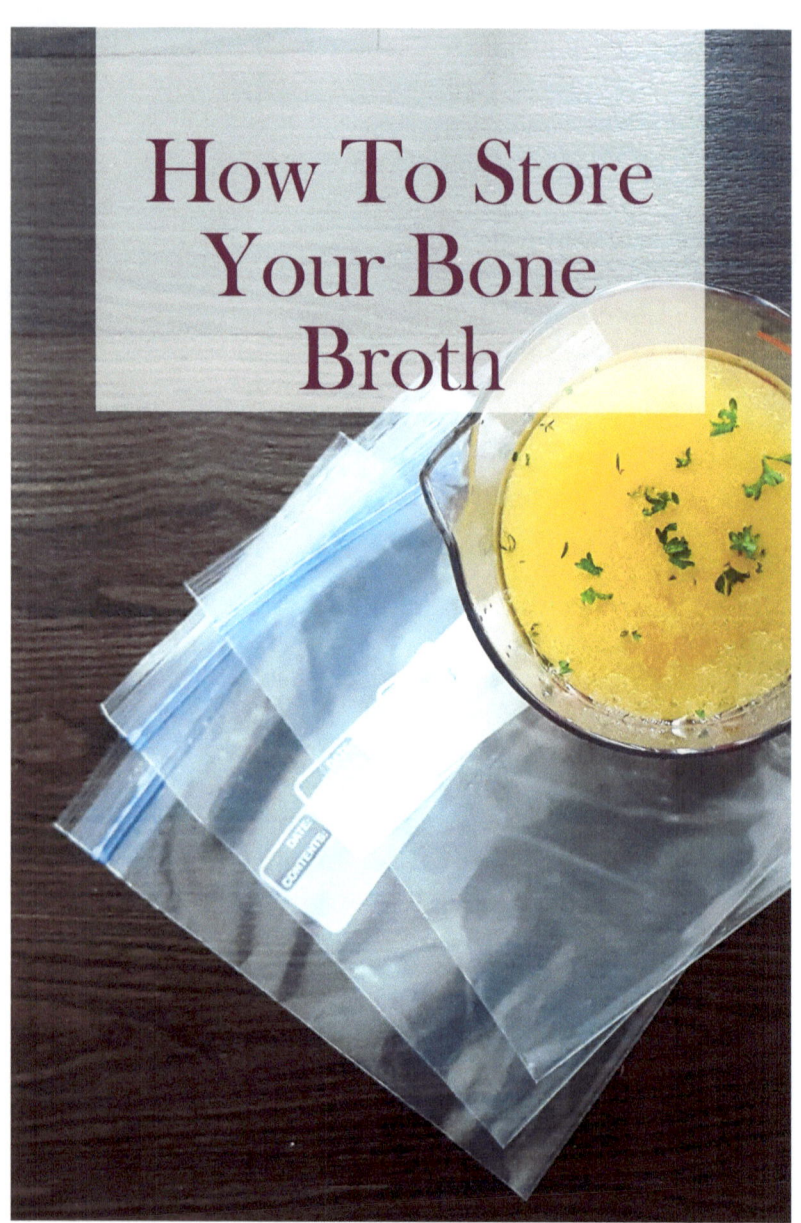

How To Store Your Bone Broth

7 HOW TO STORE YOUR BONE BROTH

Okay, you've made your first batch of bone broth and the prospect of a healthy gut, longer hair and fabulous skin (thanks to the collagen) has you dancing. The local butcher knows you by name and you're buying bones by the pound with the confidence of a multi-million-dollar CEO. But with more bones come more broth. Let's go over how to safely store your bone broth so that you may continue to enjoy it in the days to come.

Storing Bone Broth In The Fridge

Allow your bone broth to cool completely after you've finished boiling it. Anything you haven't used up by this point should be strained into clean jars and stored in the fridge for up to a week.

After your bone broth has been made, allow it to completely cool before proceeding. The last thing you want is scalding broth splashing on you as you strain it. If you are in a hurry, you can speed up the process by filling the sink halfway with ice water and placing the pot in it to cool. Then, you can store your broth in the fridge. Placing a hot pot of broth into the fridge can lower the temperature of the foods in your fridge as the heat escapes, leading to spoilage.

Once the bone broth has completely cooled in the fridge, the fat from the broth can be easily removed by carefully discarding the top layer.

Broth can readily be pulled from the fridge to add to your meals. To enjoy a cup of broth to drink, simply pour about a cup into a small pot and warm it over the stove.

Spices and herbs can also be added to taste at this time. It's a nice way to pop the flavor of a broth that has been in the fridge for a few days.

Freezing Bone Broth For Long Term Storage

If you have made more broth than you can consume within the next few days, you definitely want to freeze the balance. Once the bone broth has cooled, store about 3 days' worth in the fridge. Take the rest and immediately store in the freezer.

To avoid thawing a large portion when you only need a small amount, portion your broth before you freeze it. Individual one cup servings for drinking can easily be stored in a 1-quart freezer bag. Larger portions for meals can be stored in plastic containers or glass jars. Ice cube trays can hold broth for recipes that require smaller amounts, like flavoring vegetables and sauces. Again, use what works best for you.

Once you have decided on the container, stir the broth for even distribution and then add to your containers. Ensure the broth is cooled to room temperature before placing the containers in the freezer for storage.

Label with the date and contents and you are good to go. If you are going the ice tray route, once the broth is frozen, pop the cubes out of the tray and store them in a large freezer bag.

Because they have been individually frozen, you can now grab a few as you need without them sticking together. Cool.

PREP CHECKLIST

Ingredients

- ☐ Chicken or Turkey Bones
- ☐ Beef Bones *
- ☐ Pork Bones
- ☐ Lamb Bones *
- ☐ Apple Cider Vinegar
- ☐ Water

* Roast these bones at 450F for 20 minutes before using in the broth for the best flavor.

Optional
- ☐ Herbs and Spices
- ☐ Vegetables
  - o Onion
  - o Carrots
  - o Celery
- ☐ Salt and Pepper To Taste

Tools

- ☐ Large Stock Pot
- ☐ Strainer
- ☐ Plastic Containers, Freezer Bags, Glass Jars for Storage

Recipe:

- 3 - 4 pounds of bones
- 2 – 3 tablespoons apple cider vinegar
- 1 teaspoon salt
- 2 - 3 liters of water

Get out a large stock pot (6 quart or bigger) and put your bones in. Fill it with water and add the salt, vinegar. Cook for 12 to 48 hours.

If using vegetables add six hours prior to ending desired cook time.

Fresh herbs should be added 0-1 hour prior to ending desired cook time.

Allow the mixture to cool and strain into clean containers for storage.

Cooking Time:

- Beef, Pork, Lamb 18 to 48 Hours.
- Chicken or Poultry: 12 to 24 Hours
- Fish: 8 Hours

Storing Bone Broth

- Refrigerated for up to a week.
- Freezer for up to a year.

If you haven't tried making homemade bone broth, do yourself a favor and make your first pot this week. The flavor will surpass that of any canned or carton stock that you buy at the grocery store and you will ensure the health benefits that these shelf varieties are lacking.

It's affordable and smart in the sense that bone broth is made from the bones that you would most likely discard. And the water you'd use to cook it doesn't incur any additional cost. Even purchased bones at the store or grocer will outweigh the cost of compromised health.

There has been quite a bit of buzz surrounding bone broth but in reality, it's been healing bodies for centuries. We've reviewed the health benefits of bone broth, techniques to produce a nourishing broth and how to create a flavor that is uniquely our own.

Time to stop reading and take action to heal your gut and boost your nutritional intake. So grab a pot, pick up some bones and get work. Your gut, taste buds and checking account will thank you.

AUTHOR'S NOTE

This is just a small sample of the natural health information that I enjoy sharing on my blog.

Please visit me at www.oloxir.com for more natural health tips and home remedies.

Health & Happiness,

Marie from Oloxir